Introduction

What is Insulin Resistance?

Now that you have an idea of what is Insulin and what is its use in the body, we will see what insulin resistance is. Insulin resistance is basically a medical term that refers to a condition in which the body cells do not act normally to the hormone Insulin. Insulin is produced inside the body in pancreas. It controls the blood sugar levels in the body and regulates it as well. When the cells in the body do not respond effectively to the Insulin in pancreas, blood sugar levels rise in the body. Our brain detects this change and pancreas start producing more Insulin as a result. Due to increased production of Insulin in the body, type 2 diabetes is normally diagnosed. However it is to be kept in mind that this type of diabetes is not diagnosed in the early stages as increased Insulin production often goes unnoticed for long periods of time. One should be careful and should have regular yearly medical checkups especially those who have a history of diabetes in their family. This late detection of diabetes often causes latent autoimmune diabetes in adults. Now that you understand the term Insulin resistance, we shall have a brief look on its signs and symptoms.

Chapter 1: Understanding Insulin Resistance

History of Insulin

„Our modern, deadline-a-day lifestyle overtaxes our adrenal glands, which end up overproducing cortisol, which in turn makes it nearly impossible to sleep and can put you at risk for a heart attack. Raised cortisol also boosts your insulin levels, which can cause you to pack on the pounds, especially around the midsection."

- Suzanne Somers

Since the very first humans that walked on planet Earth, mankind has tried to make his life better with each passing day. If you travel back to the ancient times you would not survive for long. Thousands of years ago humans did not have the standard of life we have nowadays. They used to live in caves and used to eat raw meat and what not. But as the human race progressed we learned how to become more civilized. We made wonderful technological advances and hence we have such great standards of living today. The race for further advancement is still on and researchers and scientists are trying to make our live better with each passing day.

If you have a grandmother who was born in 1920s and is nearing 100, take some time out and ask her how life was in the 20' century. She will tell you all sorts of stuff. She will tell you about the time when people used candles and lanterns to light their houses at night. She may even tell you stories of the way people used to travel by ships and horse driven carriages. But among all these stories, she will tell you stories about deadly plagues and diseases. It is a known fact that the medical science was not very advanced in those times. Since we are particularly dealing with diabetics here, the condition of diabetics in those times was also very bad. People who had diabetes had very strict diet plans and there was no way to control their sugar levels. Some people even died of starvation as they could not eat a lot because of being diabetics.

It was in the year 1921 that a revolutionary drug was discovered and it was named Insulin. Two German researchers first discovered Insulin in pancreas of a dog. At that time doctors around the world did not know that Insulin was the only thing missing from a diabetic's pancreas. It was in 1910 that we discovered the real cause of diabetes. It happened because of no Insulin in pancreas. In the year 1921, a young surgeon named Federick Banting discovered a method to separate Insulin from dog's pancreas and with the help of extracted Insulin they kept a dog with diabetes alive for several days. This was the time when Insulin was truly discovered as a life changing drug.

Why Diabetics Need Insulin?

The body of a person who has diabetes does not produce enough Insulin and Amylin to control the blood sugar levels. This is the primary reason that diabetics have to take Insulin in order to survive. If someone who is a diabetic and he /she does not take Insulin, their blood sugar levels vary a lot. This is not only dangerous but it is harmful for the health as well. Consider a person who is working alone in a farm and he is a diabetic, his sugar level suddenly drops and he faints. Now this is a very dangerous situation and this can cost that person his life. To avoid all similar situations, a person suffering from diabetes has to take Insulin. Fortunately or unfortunately this is the only way for them to spend a normal life.

Symptoms of Insulin Resistance

People who have Insulin Resistance have shown various signs but they differ from person to person. Some of the signs that people with Insulin resistance normally show are:

- Difficulty in focusing
- Some people also gain a lot of weight
- Increase in appetite
- A sleepiness feeling after meals
- High levels of sugar in blood
- Depression
- Blood pressure is also known to increase

Diagnosis of Insulin Resistance

Usually the insulin level and blood glucose level while fasting tell us if a person has insulin resistance or diabetes. However, just to be sure additional tests may be performed as recommended by the doctor. For a non-diabetic person high level of blood sugar while fasting is abnormal and should be immediately acted upon by going to a health care professional and by consulting him.

If you have the above mentioned symptoms especially if you have high levels of blood sugar and you have an increased hunger, you should visit your doctor. Insulin resistance cannot be diagnosed by a common man and you require a health care professional for the proper diagnosis of Insulin Resistance. Once you pay a visit to your doctor, tell him all the signs that you feel and then let him perform some laboratory tests along with the physical examination.

Summary of Chapter 1

These are symptoms of Insulin resistance:

1. A sleepiness feeling after meals

2. High levels of sugar in blood

3. Difficulty in focusing

4. Some people also gain a lot of weight

5. Increase in appetite

6. Depression

7. Blood pressure is also known to increase

Insulin resistance cannot be diagnosed by a common man and you require a health care professional for the proper diagnosis of Insulin Resistance.

Chapter 2

Cure for Insulin Resistance

Insulin Resistance does not have a medical cure. By a medical cure we mean some medicine, injection or a surgery that can help you get rid of Insulin resistance. The only way to control insulin resistance is by changing your lifestyle. There are two ways in which changed lifestyle can help you control insulin resistance. These are:

1. Need of insulin can be controlled
2. Reaction of cells to insulin can be enhanced

Let us take a look at how the above two things can be achieved. This is basically what this book focuses on and this is what is known as body fat solution and belly fat cure. The mentioned solution focuses on a complete lifestyle change which involves a lot of exercise and controlled and healthy eating. We shall see one by one the things that can help you treat insulin resistance in the next chapter. At the moment we will focus on how the need of insulin is decreased and sensitivity of cells to insulin is increased by the body.

Lower the Need for Insulin

When you eat something it has different levels of proteins, carbohydrates, vitamins and other minerals. Eggs and meat are high protein diet while bread and potato are high carbohydrate foods. Citrus fruits contain large quantities of vitamin C and other vitamins. Sunlight is a great source of vitamin D. Now that we know that each food has varying quantities of different things, we can establish how these foods act inside our body.

If a person that is suffering from insulin resistance takes only those foods that have low carbohydrate content and the foods that have low glycemic index, he can decrease his need of insulin. But this comes over a period of time and you have to be very diet conscious. The moment you step out of the line things will start going wrong. Once you eat a controlled diet for a certain period of time, your body will get tuned to low insulin demand and you will start feeling that your insulin resistance has been cured to a certain extent.

People who have insulin resistance should particularly be considerate about taking those foods that have high carbohydrate content. It is to be mentioned that different foods that have high quantity of carbohydrates in them have different glycemic indices. Glycemic index determines how fast the carbohydrate will break down into the sugar components and then get absorbed in the blood. Those foods that have high glycemic index increase the sugar level in blood faster than those with low glycemic index.

Increased Sensitivity of Cells to Insulin

Insulin resistance as we know is mainly caused by the cells being unresponsive to the hormone insulin. Either they are unresponsive or they do not act normally to insulin. But this condition can be improved. You just need to tune your body so that the cells start to respond more properly to the hormone insulin. There are different ways to do that.

The best way to increase the sensitivity of cells is to exercise. When you exercise, your heartbeat rate increases and more blood is pumped into your body. Higher the blood flow rate, higher is the need for oxygen. In addition to that your body demands more energy when you exercise and this need for energy is compensated by the glucose present in your body. Increased glucose intake by body enhances insulin sensitivity of cells and hence with regular exercise the sensitivity of cells towards insulin can be increased.

There are certain substances that researchers have found over the years which help in curing insulin resistance. Amylomaize is one of those substances which is known to lessen insulin resistance in people who have type 2 diabetes and also in healthy individuals. There are some acids that possess some ability to restrict insulin resistance. But they are not a permanent cure and they can only moderate progression from insulin resistance to diabetes.

A lot of research has been done on various substances over the past few years and researchers have not been able to find one good substance that is a cure to insulin resistance. But research has proved one thing that eating a controlled diet and doing exercise regularly is twice as effective against insulin resistance as compared to the substances available as yet. The reason behind the effectiveness of these two things is the reduction of fat in the entire body and especially the belly. Of course this is not the only reason behind this. There are other reasons as well which have been stated above. In the upcoming chapters we will have a look at how you can help yourself

to implement the body fat solution for insulin resistance.

Summary of Chapter 2

Very important thing to remember:

<u>You can CONTROL Insulin!</u>

- Insulin resistance as we know is mainly caused by the cells being unresponsive to the hormone insulin

- People who have insulin resistance should particularly be considerate about taking those foods that have high carbohydrate content. It is to be mentioned that different foods that have high quantity of carbohydrates in them have different glycemic indices. Glycemic index determines how fast the carbohydrate will break down into the sugar components and then get absorbed in the blood.

- Once you eat a controlled diet for a certain period of time, your body will get tuned to low insulin demand and you will start feeling that your insulin resistance has been cured to a certain extent.

Chapter 3

What's The Best Diet For You?

A wise man once said that there are two things that are in your control and you can change them according to your own will. One is the amount of food you eat and second is the amount of time you sleep. Nature has made humans in such a way that they are very flexible. A human being can get used to 12 hours of sleep and he can also get used to 4 hours of sleep. Similarly human body can get used to 3,000 calories a day or it can be tuned to 1,000 calories a day. It all depends on the person. Restricting yourself to a healthy diet also depends on you. If you decide to eat all the junk in the world, no one can stop you. And if you decide to eat healthy food all the time, no one can stop you. You are your own king.

A proper diet plan can help you reduce body and belly fat and ultimately it can help you cure insulin resistance. We will see what types of food you need to eat in order to cure insulin resistance. The timing of the meals is also important. So in this chapter we will try to make a diet plan for you that can help you cure insulin resistance. Let's have a look at the types of foods that are good and that are bad for anyone suffering from insulin resistance. Let's start with the foods you should avoid.

Foods to avoid

„Carbohydrates, and especially refined ones like sugar, make you produce lots of extra insulin. I've been keeping my intake really low ever since I discovered this. I've cut out all starch such as potatoes, noodles, rice, bread and pasta."

- Cynthia K.

You have to be very careful when you eat if you are suffering from insulin resistance. Any bad choices you make will make your case worse. Insulin resistance can only be overcome with patience and by disciplining yourself. We shall now look at some foods that are really bad choices when it comes to insulin resistance.

French Fries

Potatoes are a lot of starch people! When you fry them in oil, you are making it worse for yourself. Potatoes absorb a lot of oil and hence you are eating a lot of fat and extra calories. Do not eat those French fries folks. Otherwise get ready for more problems associated with insulin resistance.

White Bread

White bread is a type of refined starch and it acts like sugar when it goes into your body. White bread is a really bad choice when it comes to insulin resistance. Do not take white bread at any cost. Prefer whole wheat bread instead which is usually brown in color.

Whole Milk

We discussed in the good food section that milk is good for insulin resistant people. But it is to be kept in mind that whole milk is a lot of fat which is not good insulin resistance. You should take low-fat milk or skimmed milk. Low-fat milk in fact is a great food for insulin resistant people.

Candy

Now that is pretty obvious. Any type of candy you eat is harmful for you as it involves direct sugar intake. Candies do not only raise the sugar level in blood but they also create complications for insulin resistant people. If you want to eat something sweet, eat a fruit or yogurt with brown sugar. Avoid candies at all possible costs.

Fruit Juices

Although the fruits are a very healthy option to eat for people who have insulin resistance but it is important to know that fruit juices are not. Even the freshly made juices are not so good for such people. The i00% fruit juice that is available in the market is also not good and they create spikes in blood sugar level.

Raisins

Raisins should not be confused with nuts. As nuts and raisin both are classified as dry fruits, many people mistake raisins as nuts. While the nuts are good for insulin resistant people, raisins are not!

Pancakes

This is the worst breakfast choice that an insulin resistant person can make. Both pancakes and syrup contain a lot of carbohydrates and cause a lot of problems in your blood sugar levels. When you have a craving for pancakes, suppress it and instead make an egg with loads of vegetables.

Bacon

Bacon is a very high fat meat. It has a lot of health disadvantages and should be avoided at all costs even by healthy individuals. As people with insulin resistance have a greater chance of heart diseases, so bacon and other high fat meat are like poison. Do not eat that bacon peeps or you will soon be in a lot of trouble.

Cakes and Snacks

All the packed snacks, cakes and pastries are full of sugar and should be avoided at all costs. They create spikes in blood sugar level and cause inflammation. Due to this insulin cannot act properly and for people who have insulin resistance, this means big problems!

Foods to Eat

„I need insulin to stay alive. It's just therapy to keep going. What I can do is make sure that I keep my blood sugar down to a reasonable level. I can exercise, and I can eat properly. And insulin plays a very big part in that."

- Mary Moore

Many people know that any type of food that has sugar in it is not good for people with diabetes or in this case insulin resistance. We will discuss here the types of foods that increase your blood sugar levels and are harmful for people suffering from insulin resistance. It is important to note that there are some other types of foods that are harmful although sugar directly is not involved in them. So here are some types of foods that are good for people with insulin resistance.

Beef

Now how many of you thought that beef is a bad food for diabetic people? You are wrong people! Beef is a friendly food for diabetics. But the condition of course is that you don't eat a lot of it. Always choose the leanest cuts and eat appropriate amount of beef. Try to cut the fat off from meat when you eat ft. If you cannot remove it easily, keep the beef in freezer for half an hour. This makes the beef a little harder and makes it easier to remove fat. Now if anyone tells you "You can't eat meat," tell them "Yes I can!"

Broccoli

That green looking vegetable isn't that bad especially if you are a diabetic. It is full of antioxidants and it is extremely fibrous. Both these things fight against insulin resistance. High quantity of chromium present in it stabilizes the sugar level in blood for long periods of time. Now don't make that face when you see Broccoli. Remember, it is good for your health.

Barley

Most of the people prefer rice. But let me tell you, if you choose barley over rice, the rise in blood sugar level after the meal cuts down by 70%. Now that is a big cut! Add barley in your soups or serve it as a side dish. Compounds present in barley slow digestion and hence the absorption of sugar in blood. Thus barley keeps your sugar level maintained.

Nuts

Nuts are another food that digests at a slow pace. They have high quantity of protein and fibre and hence are extremely good for people who have insulin resistance. They also contain large amounts of mono saturated fat that helps to reverse insulin resistance. Nuts can be added as toppings on your main serving.

Beans

Beans are an excellent source of soluble fiber. It literally puts a lid on your blood sugar level. They have a lot of protein as well and hence can serve as the main ingredient in any dish.

Berries

All types of berries are excellent for treating insulin resistance. They are rich in fibre and have a good amount of antioxidants as well. They help to control high blood sugar and are a source to reduce body fat as well.

Avocado

Avocados are full of mono saturated fats which are extremely beneficial for insulin resistance cure. They are tasty and help to keep blood sugar level in control especially after the meals. Avocados can even help you reverse insulin resistance if you take them for long periods of time.

Flaxseed

The shiny brown flaxseeds are not something you feed to the birds. This is something that is rich in fiber and good fats. Both of these things are great for treating insulin resistance. You can sprinkle the seeds on some cereal or yogurt if you don't like them as they are.

Olive Oil

Olives have so many benefits that its oil is known as liquid gold. People who take olive oil on regular basis have much less chances of diabetes and heart diseases. Unlike other oils and butter, olive oil contains good fats which help fight against insulin resistance. You can make it a habit to cook food in olive oil. This is a really good and healthy option if you have insulin resistance.

Whole-grain Bread

Most commonly available bread in the market is white bread which is extremely unhealthy for people who have insulin resistance. The reason is high carbohydrates content which produces a lot of glucose and raises the sugar level in blood. On the other hand whole-grain bread helps to improve insulin sensitivity and is great for maintaining blood sugar levels within limits. Always use whole grain bread instead of white bread. There are some types of bread available that have written on them multigrain or some other stuff like that, do not confuse them with whole grain bread. If the bread doesn't have the word "whole", do not buy i

Apple

An apple a day, keeps the doctor away. We have heard that a number of times but still we don't act upon it. Apples are very low in calories and high in fibrous content. They fulfill your appetite quickly and help to avoid peaks in blood sugar levels. Along with these things apples have a lot of other health advantages as well. Apples are most beneficial when they are eaten unpeeled. The skin of apples is extremely good for health.

Fish

We know you like seafood and fish is actually good for people who have insulin resistance. If you have insulin resistance, you have a greater chance of getting a heart disease. However if you eat fish the chance of a heart disease reduces by 4o%. Many people are of the view that it has some disadvantages as well. But the truth is that the benefits of fish outweigh its disadvantages by a huge margin.

Oatmeal

Oatmeal is a wonder food for people with insulin resistance as it contains a lot of soluble fibre which helps to slow down the process of consuming carbohydrates by the body. Hence it keeps your blood sugar level stable and decreases the need for insulin. Just what you need, isn't it?

Milk/Yogurt

Both are extremely rich in calcium and protein. Both these things can help you lose weight and reduce the fat on your body. In addition to that the dairy products help your body fight against insulin resistance. You can buy fat-free milk if you don't like the other milk. There are plenty of options available to suit your need and taste.

The Perfect Meal

Since you cannot count the number of carbohydrates

and other substances in anything and cannot look it up on the internet before every meal that you take, we discuss here the perfect meal that you can have. There are a few things that you need to keep in mind while you take your meals. These are:

- Do not eat a lot at once.
- Eat in intervals.

This increases insulin sensitivity, improves digestion and prevents you from accumulating fat.

Minimize the number of things that have a lot of carbohydrates.

Take a complete and balanced meal.

- Do not eat a lot of beef or chicken at once.
- Always take small portions of it and always combine with vegetables to fulfill your appetite.

- Learn about which pieces of meat have the lowest fat, prefer those!

GOLDEN RULE:

Choose organic products over inorganic products.

Take in a good quantity of omega-3 every week. You can get omega-3 by eating omega-3 eggs for breakfast every day.

Eat veggies that have low-glycemic indices such as broccoli, cabbage, asparagus, spinach etc.

Take small amounts of low sugar fruit every day in intervals. Some good low sugar fruit are plums, pears, cherries, apples and berries.

Include seasoning agents such as ginger, turmeric and rosemary in your food. They are excellent detoxifiers and anti-oxidants. Hence they reduce body fat and maintain blood sugar level.

Take as much fibrous food as you can.

Use olive oil to cook your food. It is the best option amongst cooking oils for insulin resistant people.

Eat nuts and seeds. If you don't like them, crush them and spread on your main dishes and you will see that they taste delicious.

Use garlic and onion in your meal.

Breakfast, Lunch and Dinner

Breakfast

Choose food that is rich in protein for breakfast. A good option is omega-3 eggs. You can also take soy protein shakes or small amount of butter with nuts. Eat a handful of almonds in the morning as well. They are a rich source of protein.

Snacks

Eat every 3-4 hours to maintain a good level of blood sugar. Do not eat a lot at once. Choose the snacks that are rich in protein. You can eat nuts, raw vegetables etc.

Lunch

Take a meal that has balanced amounts of protein, carbs and fats. Combine your main course with nuts, vegetables and fruits at lunch.

Dinner

Eat something as balanced as the lunch and make sure that you finish eating 2-3 hours before bed. Do not take bed time snacks as they may cause complications. Also bed time snacks cause accumulation of fat on belly and other parts of body.

Summary of Chapter 3

<u>If you have insulin resistance you should avoid:</u>

Candy

Fruit Juices

Raisins

Pancakes

French Fries

White Bread

Whole Milk

Bacon

Cakes and Snacks

<u>There's a list of foods that you should include in your meal plan:</u>

Beans

Berries

Avocado

Beef

Flaxseed

Olive Oil

Whole-grain Bread

Broccoli

Barley

Nuts

Yogurt and Milk

Apples

Carrots

Fish

Oatmeal

Chapter 4

Exercising is crusial

I am pretty sure that you know by now that any type of fat is poison for you if you are an insulin resistant. Insulin resistance can be overcome by disciplining yourself. We have discussed this thing time and again in the last chapters. I know that exercising regularly is not an easy job and something will always come up in your busy schedule that will make you miss exercise for the day. But hey, where there is a will, there is a way!

It is important that you make up your mind about exercising regularly. Start taking it as a vital part of your daily routine. Exercising is as important to you as your meal. If you don't eat properly, you get ill and may even die if you don't eat for too long. Now replace your food with exercise. Make yourself believe that if you don't exercise you will die! Trust me; this is the best way to fit in a proper exercise schedule.

We have discussed that insulin resistance can be overcome by taking proper food and by exercising. Now let us establish the type of exercise you need to do in order to effectively burn the fats and carbohydrates that you take in. The timings of the exercise are also important. Let us see what the best times are and what the best exercises are in those times that you can do in order to burn fat and get control over insulin resistance.

Walking

Make a schedule so that you can get up early. Do not stay awake at night as this will make you crave for snacks which are bad for your health. In addition to that you will be able to get up early in the morning for the early morning walk. If you have a job due to which you can't or you are too lazy to get up early in the morning, just go on a walk when you wake up without eating anything. Drink a glass of water before you go on the walk or take a water bottle with you so that you don't feel thirsty.

If you are young enough to jog or run, I would say you jog. When you are on an empty stomach and you go on a walk or a jog, your body takes energy from the food that you ate at night or from the fats that have accumulated inside your body. This is one of the best ways to burn body fat. Morning walks are very effective at controlling insulin levels and you will see that your insulin resistance will decrease. I would recommend that you keep a handful of almonds in your pocket in case your blood sugar level drops while you are on a jog.

Another important thing to keep in mind is that you don't over exert. Just do as much walk or jog as you easily can. This walk need you to keep cardiac rhythm controlled to maximize effect and for sure, you don't want to faint by a decrease in your blood sugar level now, do you? It's vital to take breakfast immediately after the walk to help body to recover itself.

Yoga / Stretching

There are numerous videos and tutorials available on the internet that teach you how to do Yoga. Yoga is really effective in the morning as you are on an empty stomach. One good thing about yoga is that you breathe deep. This helps to improve your digestive and respiratory system. Yoga is known to reduce fat on your body very quickly and is a really good option if you want to get slim and control your insulin resistance.

Gym Time

Always take some time out for exercising in the evening. The best time to do exercise is after 2-3 hours of lunch as all the food that you have eaten at lunch is broken down into the components by now and has been absorbed by your body. This is the time when the blood sugar levels are at their maximum. If you study human biology a little, you will notice that fats also accumulate in the body during this time. Hence this is the best time to prevent fat from accumulating inside your body and also to burn the existing fats in your body. Let us have a look at how you can do this.

If you do exercises specifically related to the part of body where fats are present, you will only be preventing the accumulation of additional fats. Plus of course these exercises will strengthen your muscles. But in order to remove the already existing fat, you need to combine strength workouts with cardio. This is the best way to burn fat on your body. Let us take a look at how you can combine strength workout with cardio. Another important thing is the interval time between exercises and we shall cover that too in the next section.

Strength training and Cardio

There are a few things that you need to understand before you start your strength and cardio workouts. Strength training will build your muscles and will make them lean. Lean muscles prevent fat from accumulating on them as they immediately burn the fat that comes their way. Strength workouts also make your muscles stronger and give a nice shape to your body.

Now consider a muscle that is already under a lot of fat. Strength training will make them grow and keep burning fat while resting. In addition to that to burn fat you need to do some aerobic exercises. Cardio workouts increase the blood flow rate and make your heart stronger. Remember that a healthy heart is really important if you have insulin resistance. It will lower the chances of you getting a heart disease.

Now we move on to how to combine strength and cardio workouts. If you go on the interne and search about these workouts you will see a debate about whether strength workout should be performed before cardio or you should workout the other way around. Different people will have different opinions. I would recommend doing strength and cardio on alternate days of the week. This is the best solution in my view especially for people who have insulin resistance.

If you do both the workouts on the same day and even if you do a small amount of cardio and a small amount of strength, chances are you will get tired a lot and you won't be able to cope up with it considering your insulin resistance problem. In addition to that they won't be as effective either. If you do cardio on day 1 and focus all your energy on it and then on day 2 you do strength workout, you will yield much better results. If you don't find it suitable, you can do both the workouts on the same day. Since you need to burn the already present fat first, I would recommend doing cardio workout first.

Summary of Chapter 4

Incorporating these things into your daily routine will benefit you greatly:

- Yoga

- Stretching

- Low intensity Cardio

- High intensity Cardio (or HIIT)

- Weight Lifting

- Walking or light jog

It is important that you make up your mind about exercising regularly. Start taking it as a vital part of your daily routine. Exercising is as important to you as your meal. If you don't eat properly, you get ill and may even die if you don't eat for too long. Now replace your food with exercise.

Bonus Videos!

Let's make this interesting! I've decided to add videos in this book, in my opinion, you will benefit greatly from them, improve your overall health and expand your horizons.

https://www.youtube.com/watch?v=rwnonffgvM0

https://www.youtube.com/watch?v=5-ThdyK4_x4

https://www.youtube.com/watch?v=cAyoiCe-OO0

Huge Thank You!

First and foremost, Thank You for downloading this book. At the end of the day I'm **extremely** grateful for **every** download and **every** purchase. It really makes me smile and motivates me. I wish that every person would put their best forward for the human race. I wish you unlimited mental strength and discipline to achieve your goals and dreams. **Together** we can make the difference.

If you found the information useful I would be extremely grateful if you could write a short Amazon review. It really does make the difference and I personally read every review and take notes. I want to improve my books, so that I can provide more value to other people. I know that my future books will give you the best experience possible.

Copyright

Disclaimer